The Complete Bread Machine Cooking Guide

Quick And Easy Bread Maker Recipes For Beginners

Jude Lamb

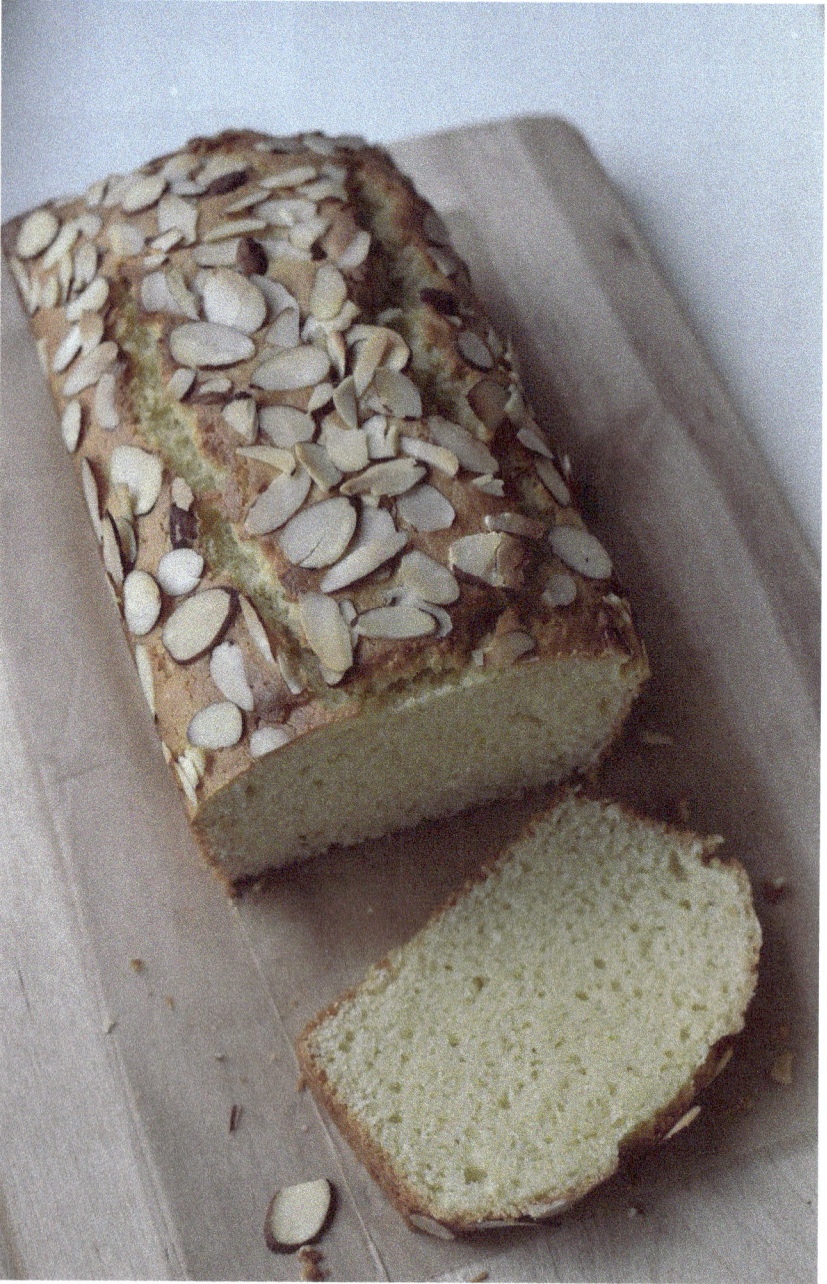

Table of contents

Making Bread

There is nothing like the scent of freshly baked bread to greet you when you wake up. Bakers traditionally produced their products during the early hours meaning their loaves were fresh, hot, and mouth-watering tasty for hungry customers wanting a slice of bread to go with a slap-up breakfast.

Bread historically dates back to Neolithic or even prehistoric times in its earliest incarnation.

Prime ingredients include flour and water used to make the dough. The dough can have numerous additives to offer assorted consistency, flavors, and healthy preferences. Additives may include yeast, fat, salt, baking soda, fruits, spices, eggs, milk, sugar, or vegetables. You can even add seeds to the bread, oils, and nuts. Bread is quite a versatile product and can be devoured on its own or as an accompaniment to the main dish. The dough is traditionally baked, but modern alternatives could include steaming.

The outer part of the bread, commonly known as the crust, can be baked into a hard or soft version. The inner part of the bread is classed as the "crumb," strangely not the small bits that cover your lap.

The prime time to eat a loaf of bread is soon after it has been removed from the oven. At this delicious time, the bread is warm, aromatic, and fresh. Leaving the bread for any length of time will cause the bread to become stale.

A quirk dating back to the 13th century was the Baker's Dozen.

A Baker's Dozen, ironic as it was from the 13th century, relates to 13 items making a dozen instead of the usual 1 1/2. As history would have us believe, a Baker's dozen suggested that punishment was administered to bakers who short-changed their customers. One way to ensure that a customer always received a full quota was to give more bread than paid for. Furthermore, if one loaf was damaged, burnt or was of unacceptable quality, there were still 1 1/2 loaves available for the customer.

Another explanation of the Baker's Dozen, and slightly more believable, is that when round loaves were placed on a standard baking tray, the configuration was 3+2+3+2+3 which gave a greater density to the tray and allowed easier stacking.

Over the decades, the baking of bread has followed the path of many traditions updated to reflect the changing needs of society. Whereas bread was always the preserve of the local baker, modern supermarkets now have their own "in-house" ovens, and bread is baked to suit customer demand.

Avocado Pancakes for keto diet

Preparation Time: 5 minutes

Cooking time: 10 minutes

Servings: 4

Ingredients:

- 1 large avocado
- 2 eggs
- ½ cup milk
- ¼ cup almond flour
- ½ teaspoon baking powder
- 1 tablespoon erythritol

Directions:

1. Mix all ingredients in a blender.
2. Preheat a skillet and coat with non-stick spray.
3. Ladle in the batter and cook for 1-2 minutes per side.

Nutrition:

- Kcal per serve: 199
- Fat:: 16 g. (70%)
- Protein: 7 g. (16%)
- Carbohydrates: 7 g. (14%)

Healthy Almond Bars

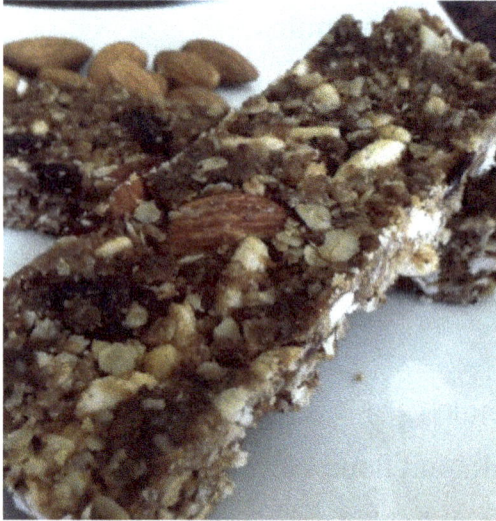

Preparation Time: 10 minutes

Cooking time: 25 minutes

Servings: 6

Ingredients:

- 2 large eggs
- 1/2 teaspoon vanilla
- 2 1/2 tablespoons swerve
- 2 tablespoons almond butter
- ½ cup of coconut oil
- ¼ cup coconut flour
- 1 ½ cup almond flour

- Pinch of salt

Directions:

Pour 1 cup of water into the instant pot, then place a trivet in the pot.

Add all the ingredients into a food processor and process until well combined.

Take one baking pan which fits into your instant pot. Line the baking pan with parchment paper.

Add dough to the pan and spread dough gently with the palm of your hands.

Place baking pan on top of the trivet in the instant pot.

Seal the instant pot with the lid and select manual and set the timer for 15 minutes.

Allow releasing pressure naturally for 10 minutes, then release using the quick release method.

Open the lid carefully. Remove the baking pan from the instant pot and let it cool for 20 minutes.

Slice into bars and place in the refrigerator for 1-2 hours.

Nutrition:

- Calories: 379

- Fat: 36.9 g

- Carbohydrates: 8.3 g

- Protein: 9.3 g

Berry Mousse

Preparation Time: 10 minutes

Cooking time: 16 minutes

Servings: 3

Ingredients:

- 1 cup strawberries, chopped
- 1 cup raspberries
- ¼ teaspoon ground ginger
- 1 teaspoon vanilla
- ¼ cup heavy cream
- 3 tablespoons whipped cream
- 1 cup unsweetened almond milk
- ¼ cup Swerve
- Pinch of salt

Directions:

1. Add berries, ¼ cup water, and swerve into the instant pot and cook on sauté mode for 10-12 minutes. Stir constantly and mash lightly.
2. Once most of the liquid has evaporated from the berries mixture, add the almond milk and vanilla. Stir well and cook for 3-4 minutes more.

3. Stir in heavy cream, whipped cream, ginger, and salt.

4. Transfer mousse mixture to the serving bowls and place in the refrigerator for 3-4 hours.

5. Serve chilled and enjoy.

Nutrition:

- Calories: 133

- Fat: 9.9 g

- Carbohydrates: 10.4 g

- Protein: 1.7 g

Creamy Chocolate Mousse

Preparation Time: 10 minutes
Cooking time: 20 minutes
Servings: 5

Ingredients:
- 4 egg yolks
- ½ teaspoon vanilla
- ½ cup unsweetened almond milk
- 1 cup heavy whipping cream
- ¼ cup unsweetened cocoa powder
- ¼ cup of water
- ½ cup Swerve
- Pinch of salt

Directions:
1. Add egg into a medium bowl and whisk until beaten.
2. In a saucepan, add cocoa, swerve, and water, and heat over medium heat until well combined.
3. Add almond milk and cream to the pan and whisk to combine. Just heat up the mixture and remove it from the heat. Do not boil.
4. Add vanilla and salt and mix well.

5. Slowly, pour the chocolate mixture into the egg mixture and beat constantly until well combined.
6. Pour mixture into the greased ramekins.
7. Pour 2 cups of water into the instant pot, then place a trivet in the pot.
8. Place ramekins on top of the trivet.
9. Seal pot with the lid, select manual, and set timer for 6 minutes.
10. Release pressure using the Quick-release method, then open the lid.
11. Remove ramekins from the pot and let them cool completely.
12. Place in refrigerator for 4-6 hours.
13. Serve chilled and enjoy.

Nutrition:

- Calories: 141
- Fat: 13.4 g
- Carbohydrates: 3.9 g
- Protein: 3.6 g

Ricotta Lemon Cheesecake

Preparation Time: 10 minutes

Cooking time: 30 minutes

Servings: 6

Ingredients:

- 2 eggs
- 1 lemon zest
- 1/3 cup ricotta cheese
- 1/4 cup Truvia
- 8 oz. cream cheese
- 1/2 teaspoon lemon extract
- 1 lemon juice

Directions:

1. Add all the ingredients except the eggs into the mixing bowl and using a hand mixer blend well until no lumps.
2. Add eggs and beat until well combined.
3. Pour batter into a 6-inch spring-form pan and cover with foil.
4. Pour 2 cups of water into the instant pot and place trivet into the pot.
5. Place cake pan on top of the trivet.
6. Seal pot with lid and cook on high pressure for 30 minutes.

7. Allow releasing pressure naturally, then open the lid.

8. Remove the cake pan from the pot and let it cool completely.

9. Place in the refrigerator for 5-6 hours.

10. Serve and enjoy.

Nutrition:

- Calories: 178

- Fat: 15.8 g

- Carbohydrates: 6 g

- Protein: 6.4 g

Coconut Bars

Preparation Time: 10 minutes

Cooking time: 15 minutes

Servings: 6

Ingredients:

- 3 large eggs
- 1 teaspoon vanilla
- 2 cups shredded coconut
- ¼ cup almonds, chopped
- 1 tablespoon chia seeds
- 2 tablespoons swerve
- 2 tablespoons almond butter
- ½ cup of coconut oil
- ¼ cup flaxseed meal
- Pinch of salt

Directions:

1. Pour 2 cups of water into the instant pot, then place a trivet in the pot.
2. Line a baking pan with parchment paper and set it aside.
3. Add all ingredients into the large mixing bowl and mix until the mixture is sticky.

4. Add the mixture to the prepared baking pan and spread evenly with the palms of your hands.

5. Cover baking pan with foil and place on top of the trivet in the instant pot.

6. Seal pot with the lid and select manual and set timer for 15 minutes.

7. Release pressure using the quick-release method, then open the lid.

8. Cut the bar into slices and place in the refrigerator for 1-2 hours.

Nutrition:

- Calories: 376

- Fat: 36.4 g

- Carbohydrates: 8.4 g

- Protein: 7.2 g

Chia Nut Bars

Preparation Time: 10 minutes

Cooking time: 25 minutes

Servings: 10

Ingredients:

- 1 cup almond butter
- 2 ½ tablespoons swerve
- 2 tablespoons chia seeds
- ¼ teaspoon cinnamon
- ½ cup almond flour
- ¼ cup unsweetened cocoa powder
- ¼ cup hazelnuts, chopped
- 1 cup almonds, chopped
- Pinch of salt

Directions:

1. Line a baking dish with parchment paper and set it aside.
2. Pour 1 cup of water into the instant pot and place trivet in the pot.
3. Add the almond butter, swerve, cinnamon, almond flour, cocoa powder, hazelnuts, almonds, and salt into the food processor and process until smooth.

4. Transfer mixture into the large bowl. Add chia seeds and mix well.
5. Transfer mixture into the prepared baking dish and spread mixture evenly.
6. Cover baking dish with foil and place on top of the trivet in the instant pot.
7. Seal pot with the lid and select manual and set timer for 15 minutes.
8. Allow releasing pressure naturally for 10 minutes, then release using the Quick release method.
9. Open the lid carefully. Remove the baking dish from the instant pot and let it cool for 20 minutes.
10. Cut the bar into slices and serve.

Nutrition:

- Calories. 122
- Fat: 10.3 g
- Carbohydrates: 5.9 g
- Protein: 4.6 g

Chocolate Cheesecake

Preparation Time: 10 minutes

Cooking time: 35 minutes

Servings: 6

Ingredients:

- 16 oz cream cheese
- 2 large eggs
- 4 tablespoons unsweetened cocoa powder
- 2 tablespoons heavy whipping cream
- ½ teaspoon vanilla
- 2 teaspoons coconut flour
- ½ cup Swerve

For topping:

- 2 teaspoons swerve
- ½ cup sour cream

Directions:

1. Grease spring-form pan with butter and line with parchment paper. Set aside.
2. Add cream cheese, cocoa powder, whipping cream, vanilla, coconut flour, and swerve into the large bowl and mix until well combined using a hand mixer.

3. Add eggs one at a time and mix until well combined.
4. Pour cheesecake batter into the prepared pan.
5. Pour 1 ½ cups of water into the instant pot, then place a trivet in the pot.
6. Place cake pan on top of the trivet.
7. Seal pot with the lid and cook on manual high pressure for 35 minutes.
8. Allow releasing pressure naturally and then open the lid. Remove the cake pan from the pot and let it cool completely.
9. Mix together the topping ingredients and spread them on top of the cake.
10. Place cake in the refrigerator for 3-4 hours.
11. Slice and serve.

Nutrition:

- Calories: 376
- Fat: 35.1 g
- Carbohydrates: 7.9 g
- Protein: 9.9 g

Pull-Apart Bread Rolls

Preparation Time: 2 hours

Cooking time: 15 minutes

Servings: 8

Ingredients:

- 2 cups almond flour

- 3 tablespoons psyllium husk powder

- 2 teaspoons baking powder

- 3 tablespoons whey protein powder

- 2 teaspoons insulin

- 2 teaspoons active dry yeast

- 2 egg whites

- 2 eggs

- ¼ cup butter

- 1/3 cup lukewarm water

- ¼ cup Greek yoghurt

Directions:

1. Add all ingredients to the Bread Machine.

2. Select Dough setting. When the time is over, transfer the dough to the floured surface. Shape it into a ball and then cut it into about 8 even pieces.

3. Line a pie dish with parchment paper. Form 8 dough balls. Cover the dish with greased cling film and let them sit for 60 minutes in a warm place.

4. Heat the oven to 350°F and bake for 15 minutes. Cover with foil and bake for 10 more minutes.

Nutrition:

- Calories: 257

- Fat: 20.1g

- Total carbohydrates: 7.1 g

- Protein: 12.4 g

Fluffy Paleo Bread

Preparation Time: 10 minutes

Cooking time: 40 minutes

Servings: 15

Ingredients:

- 1 ¼ cup almond flour
- 5 eggs
- 1 teaspoon lemon juice
- 1/3 cup avocado oil
- 1 dash black pepper
- ½ teaspoon sea salt
- 3 to 4 tablespoons tapioca flour
- 1 to 2 teaspoons poppy seed
- ¼ cup ground flaxseed
- ½ teaspoon baking soda

Top with:

- Poppy seeds
- Pumpkin seeds

Directions:

1. Preheat the oven to 350°F.
2. Line a baking pan with parchment paper and set it aside.

3. In a bowl, add eggs, avocado oil, and lemon juice and whisk until combined.
4. In another bowl, add tapioca flour, almond flour, baking soda, flaxseed, black pepper, and poppy seed. Mix.
5. Add the lemon juice mixture into the flour mixture and mix well.
6. Add the batter into the prepared loaf pan and top with extra pumpkin seeds and poppy seeds.
7. Cover loaf pan and transfer into the prepared oven.
8. Bake for 20 minutes. Remove cover and bake until an inserted knife comes out clean—after about 15 to 20 minutes.
9. Remove from oven and cool.
10. Slice and serve.

Nutrition:
- Calories: 149
- Fat: 12.9 g
- Carbohydrates: 4.4 g
- Protein: 5 g

Spicy Bread

Preparation Time: 10 minutes

Cooking time: 40 minutes

Servings: 6

Ingredients:

- ½ cup coconut flour
- 6 eggs
- 3 large jalapenos, sliced
- 4 ounces turkey bacon, sliced
- ½ cup ghee
- ¼ teaspoon baking soda
- ¼ teaspoon salt
- ¼ cup water

Directions:

1. Preheat the oven to 400°F.
2. Cut bacon and jalapenos on a baking tray and roast for 10 minutes.
3. Flip and bake for 5 more minutes.
4. Remove seeds from the jalapenos.
5. Place jalapenos and bacon slices in a food processor and blend until smooth.
6. In a bowl, add ghee, eggs, and ¼-cup water. Mix well.

7. Then add the coconut flour, baking soda, and salt. Stir to mix.
8. Add bacon and jalapeno mix.
9. Grease the loaf pan with ghee.
10. Pour batter into the loaf pan.
11. Bake for 40 minutes.
12. Enjoy.

Nutrition:

- Calories: 240
- Fat: 20 g
- Carbohydrates: 5 g
- Protein: 9 g

Moist Mango Bread

Preparation Time: 30 minutes
Cooking time: 55-60 minutes
Servings: 8-10 slices

Ingredients:

- 2 cups almond flour, finely ground
- 1/2 cup semi-sweet chocolate chips
- 2-3 ripe mangoes
- 1 1/4 cup toasted macadamia nuts/pecans, coarsely chopped
- 3/8 cup unsalted butter, melted
- 1/4 cup sweetener: xylitol or a combination of 1/4 cup erythritol and 1/4 cup xylitol
- 3 large eggs, lightly beaten
- 1 tablespoon baking powder
- 4 tablespoons plain full-fat yogurt or coconut milk
- 1 teaspoon baking soda
- 1 teaspoon vanilla extract

Directions:

1. Add all ingredients to the Bread Machine.

2. Select Dough setting and press Start. Mix the ingredients for about 4-5 minutes. After that press the Stop button.

3. Smooth out the top of the loaf. Choose Bake mode and press Start. Let it bake for about 55 minutes.

4. Remove bread from the bread machine and let it rest for 10 minutes. Enjoy!

Nutrition:

- Calories: 380

- Fat: 11 g

- Total carbohydrates: 46 g

- Protein: 5 g

Fluffy Cloud Bread

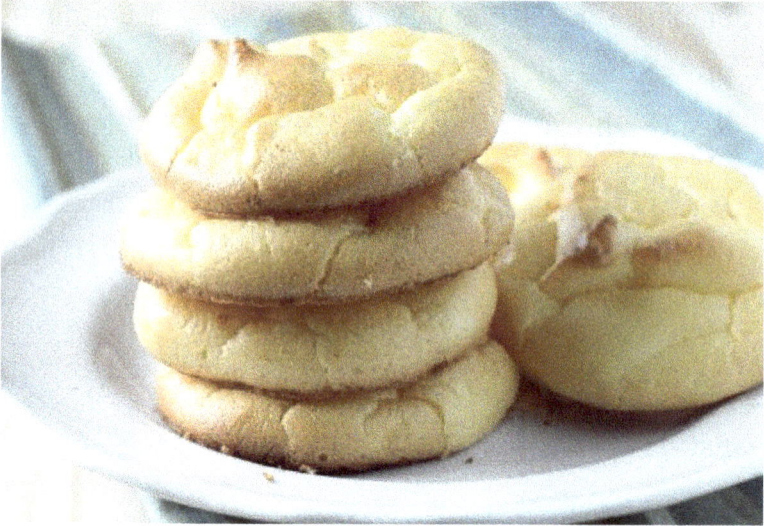

Preparation Time: 25 minutes

Cooking time: 25 minutes

Servings: 3

Ingredients:

- 1 pinch salt
- ½ tablespoon ground psyllium husk powder
- ½ tablespoon baking powder
- ¼ teaspoon cream of tarter
- 2 eggs, separated

- ½ cup, cream cheese

Directions:

1. Preheat the oven to 300°F and line a baking tray with parchment paper.
2. Whisk egg whites in a bowl until soft peaks are formed.
3. Mix egg yolks with cream cheese, salt, cream of tartar, psyllium husk powder, and baking powder in a bowl.
4. Add the egg whites carefully and transfer to the baking tray.
5. Place in the oven and bake for 25 minutes.
6. Remove from the oven and serve.

Nutrition:

- Calories: 185
- Fat: 16.4 g
- Carbohydrates: 3.9 g
- Protein: 6.6 g

Yeast Loaf Bread for keto diet

Preparation Time: 5 minutes

Cooking time: 4 hours

Servings: 16 slices (1 slice per serving)

Ingredients:

1 package dry yeast

½ teaspoon sugar

1 1/8 cup warm water about 90-100 ° F

3 tablespoons olive oil or avocado oil

1 cup vital wheat gluten flour

¼ cup oat flour

¾ cup soy flour

¼ cup flax meal

¼ cup wheat bran course, unprocessed

1 tablespoon sugar

1 ½ teaspoon baking powder

1 teaspoon salt

Directions:

1. Mix the sugar, water, and yeast in the bread bucket to try the yeast. If the yeast does not bubble, toss and replace it.

2. Combine all the dry ingredients in a bowl and mix thoroughly. Pour over the wet ingredients in the bread bucket.
3. Set the bread machine and select Basis cycle to bake the loaf. Close the lid. This takes 3 to 4 hours.
4. When the cycle ends, remove the bread from the bread machine.
5. Cool on a rack before slicing.
6. Serve with butter or light jam.

Nutrition:

- Calories: 99
- Calories from fat: 45
- Total Fat: 5 g
- Total Carbohydrates: 7 g
- Net Carbohydrates: 5 g
- Protein: 9 g

Protein Bread

Preparation Time: 10 minutes

Cooking time: 40 minutes

Servings: 12

Ingredients:

- 1/2 cup unflavored protein powder
- 6 tablespoons almond flour
- 5 pastured eggs, separated
- 1 tablespoon coconut oil
- 1 teaspoon baking powder
- 1 teaspoon xanthan gum
- 1 pinch Himalayan pink salt
- 1 pinch stevia (optional)

Direction:

1. Start by preheating the oven to 325 °F.
2. Grease a ceramic loaf dish with coconut oil and layer it with parchment paper.
3. Add egg whites to a bowl and beat well until it forms peaks.
4. In a separate bowl, mix the dry ingredients together.
5. Mix wet ingredients in another bowl and beat well.
6. Add dry mixture and mix well until smooth.
7. Add the egg whites and mix evenly.

8. Spread the bread batter in the prepared loaf pan.

9. Bake the bread for 40 minutes or until it's done.

10. Slice into 12 slices and serve.

Nutrition:

- Calories: 165
- Total Fat: 14 g
- Saturated Fat: 7 g
- Total Carbohydrates: 6 g
- Fiber: 3 g
- Protein: 5 g

Hawaiian Dinner Bread

Preparation Time: 10 minutes
Cooking time: 29 minutes
Servings: 10

Ingredients:

- 1 ½ cups almond flour
- 2 teaspoons baking powder
- 3/4 cup powdered Swerve
- 3 cups mozzarella cheese, shredded
- 3 ounces cream cheese
- 2 eggs
- 6 drops avocado oil
- 1 teaspoon fresh ginger paste

Directions:

1. Start by adding almond flour, Swerve, and baking powder to a medium-size bowl and mix together.
2. In a separate bowl, add cream cheese and mozzarella cheese and heat for 1 minute in a microwave until melted.
3. Mix well and pour this mixture into the dry mixture.
4. Whisk well, then add ginger, oil, and eggs.
5. Beat well to make a smooth, sticky dough.

6. Cut the dough into 10 equal parts.

7. Roll each piece into a ball and place them in a greased baking pan.

8. Bake them for 29 minutes or until golden brown.

9. Serve warm.

Nutrition:

- Calories: 151
- Total Fat: 12.2 g
- Saturated Fat: 2.4 g
- Cholesterol: 110 mg
- Sodium: 276 mg
- Total Carbohydrates: 3.2 g
- Fiber: 1.9 g
- Sugar: 0.4 g
- Protein: 8.8 g

Ketogenic Almond Bread

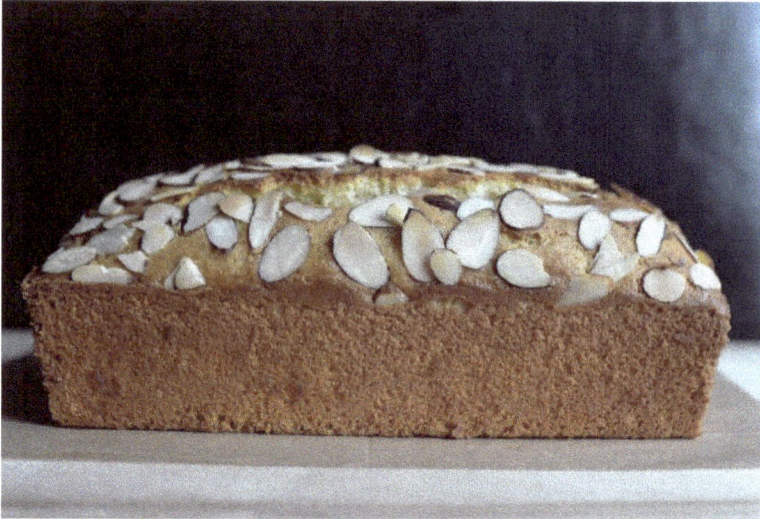

Preparation Time: 10 minutes

Cooking time: 55 min

Servings: 7

Ingredients:

- ½ cup spread
- 2 tablespoons coconut oil
- 7 eggs
- 2 cups almond flour

Directions:

1. Preheat the broiler to 355 °F.

2. Line a portion container with material paper.
3. Blend the eggs in a bowl on high for as long as two minutes.
4. Add the almond flour, liquefied coconut oil, and dissolved spread to the eggs. Keep on blending.
5. Scratch the blend into the portion container.
6. Heat for 45-50 minutes or until a toothpick comes out clean.

Nutrition:

- Calories: 21 g

- Fat: 4.7 g

- Carbohydrates: 44.2 g

- Protein: 0 g

Olive Ketogenic Bread

Preparation Time: 10 minutes
Cooking time: 25 minutes
Servings: 8

Ingredients:

- 3 tablespoons olive oil
- 2 garlic cloves, smashed
- 1¼ cups blanched almond flour
- 1 tablespoon coconut flour
- 2 teaspoons lemon zest
- 2 teaspoons baking powder
- 2 teaspoons Za'atar, divided
- ¼ teaspoon sea salt
- 1 tablespoon apple cider vinegar
- 3 large egg whites
- ½ cup shredded Mozzarella cheese
- ¼ cup Kalamata olives, pitted, chopped
- ½ cup grated Parmesan cheese

Directions:

1. Start by preheating the oven at 400 °F. Then grease a 9-inch loaf pan.

2. Put a suitable skillet over low heat and add oil and garlic to sauté for 4 minutes. Remove the garlic from the oil.

3. Whisk almond flour with lemon zest, coconut flour, baking powder, salt, and a teaspoon of Za'atar in a large bowl.

4. Mix 3 tablespoons of warm water with vinegar in a separate small bowl.

5. Beat egg whites until foamy using a hand mixer.

6. Add vinegar mixture, dry mixture, and 2 tablespoons garlic oil.

7. Mix well and add olives and mozzarella.

8. Make a smooth dough and keep it aside.

9. Mix 1 teaspoon Za'atar and Parmesan in a medium bowl.

10. Roll the dough into the Parmesan mixture and then divide the dough into small pieces.

11. Place the pieces on the baking sheet and bake for 20 minutes until golden.

12. Serve fresh.

Nutrition:

- Calories: 267
- Total Fat: 24.5 g
- Saturated Fat: 17.4 g

- Cholesterol: 153 mg
- Sodium: 217 mg
- Total Carbohydrates: 8.4 g
- Sugar: 2.3 g
- Fiber: 1.3 g
- Protein: 3.1 g

Ketogenic Blueberry Bread

Preparation Time: 10 minutes

Cooking time: 50 minutes

Servings: 8

Ingredients:

- 5 medium eggs
- 2 cups almond flour
- 2 tablespoons coconut flour
- 1/2 cup blueberries
- 1 1/2 teaspoons baking powder
- 3 tablespoons heavy whipping cream
- 1/2 cup erythritol
- 3 tablespoons butter softened
- 1 teaspoon vanilla extract

Directions:

1. Start by preheating the oven to 350 °F. Then, line a 9x 5-inch loaf pan with parchment paper and butter.
2. Whisk eggs with vanilla extract and sweetener in a large bowl using a hand mixer.
3. Once it's frothy, add whipping cream and mix well.

4. Separately, mix the dry and wet ingredients in two bowls, then whisk them together.
5. Add butter and beat well, then add the berries.
6. Evenly spread the batter in the loaf pan and bake for 50 minutes until golden brown.
7. Slice and serve.

Nutrition:

- Calories: 201

- Total Fat: 2.2 g

- Saturated Fat: 2.4 g

- Total Carbohydrates: 4.3 g

- Fiber: 0.9 g

- Protein: 8.8 g

Herbed Garlic Bread

Preparation Time: 10 minutes

Cooking time: 45 minutes

Servings: 10

Ingredients:

- ½ cup coconut flour
- 8 tablespoons melted butter, cooled
- teaspoon baking powder
- 6 large eggs
- 1 teaspoon garlic powder
- 1 teaspoon rosemary, dried
- ¼ teaspoon salt
- ½ teaspoon onion powder

Directions:

1. Prepare bread machine loaf pan, greasing it with cooking spray.
2. In a bowl, add coconut flour, baking powder, onion, garlic, rosemary, and salt into a bowl. Combine and mix well.
3. In another bowl, add eggs, and beat until bubbly on top.
4. Add melted butter into the bowl with the eggs and beat until mixed.

5. Following the instructions on your machine's manual, mix the dry ingredients into the wet ingredients and pour in the bread machine loaf pan, taking care to follow how to mix in the baking powder.
6. Place the bread pan in the machine, and select the Basic bread setting, together with the bread size and crust type, if available, then press start once you have closed the lid of the machine.
7. When the bread is ready, using oven mitts, remove the bread pan from the machine.
8. Let it cool before slicing.
9. Cool, slice, and enjoy.

Nutrition:

- Calories: 147
- Fat: 12.5 g
- Carbohydrates: 3.5 g
- Protein: 4.6 g

Flax Seed Bread

Preparation Time: 10 minutes

Cooking time: 20 minutes

Servings: 6

Ingredients:

- 2 cups flax seed, ground
- 1 tablespoon baking powder
- 1 ½ cups protein isolate
- A pinch of salt
- 6 egg whites, whisked
- 1 egg, whisked
- ¾ cup water
- 3 tablespoons coconut oil, melted
- ¼ cup stevia

Directions:

1. In a bowl, mix all dry ingredients and stir well.
2. In a separate bowl, mix the egg whites and the rest of the wet ingredients, stir well and combine the 2 mixtures.
3. Stir the bread and mix well. Pour into a loaf pan and bake at 350 °F for 20 minutes.
4. Cool the bread down, slice, and serve.

Nutrition:

- Calories: 263

- Fat: 17 g

- Fiber: 4 g

- Carbohydrates: 2 g

- Protein 20 g

Ketogenic Spinach Bread

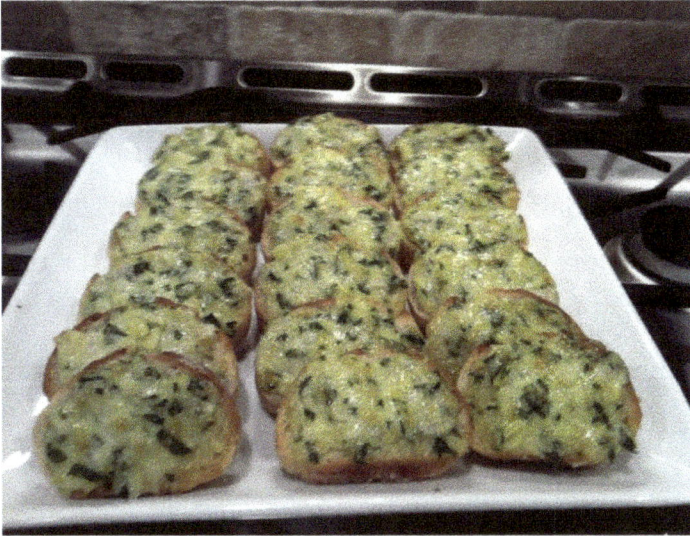

Preparation Time: 10 minutes

Cooking time: 30 minutes

Servings: 10

Ingredients:

- ½ cup spinach, chopped
- 1 tablespoon olive oil
- 1 cup water
- 3 cups almond flour
- A pinch of salt and black pepper
- 1 tablespoon stevia
- 1 teaspoon baking powder

- 1 teaspoon baking soda
- ½ cup cheddar, shredded

Directions:

1. In a bowl, mix the flour, with salt, pepper, stevia, baking powder, baking soda, and Cheddar and stir well.
2. Add the remaining ingredients, stir the batter really well and pour it into a lined loaf pan.
3. Cook at 350 °F for 30 minutes, cool the bread down, slice, and serve.

Nutrition:

- Calories: 142
- Fat: 7 g
- Fiber: 3 g
- Carbohydrates: 5 g
- Protein: 6 g

Cinnamon Asparagus Bread

Preparation Time: 10 minutes

Cooking time: 45 minutes

Servings: 8

Ingredients:

- 1 cup stevia
- ¾ cup coconut oil, melted
- 1 and ½ cups almond flour
- 2 eggs, whisked
- A pinch of salt
- 1 teaspoon baking soda
- 1 teaspoon cinnamon powder
- 2 cups asparagus, chopped
- Cooking spray

Directions:

1. In a bowl, mix all the ingredients except the cooking spray and stir the batter really well.
2. Pour this batter into a loaf pan greased with cooking spray and bake at 350 °F for 45 minutes, cool the bread down, slice, and serve.

Nutrition:

- Calories: 165

- Fat: 6 g

- Fiber: 3 g

- Carbohidrates: 5 g

- Protein: 6 g

Kale And Cheese Bread

Preparation Time: 10 minutes

Cooking time: 1 hour

Servings: 8

Ingredients:

- 2 cups kale, chopped
- 1 cup warm water
- 1 teaspoon baking powder
- 1 teaspoon baking soda
- 2 tablespoons olive oil
- 2 teaspoons stevia
- 1 cup Parmesan, grated
- 3 cups almond flour
- A pinch of salt
- 1 egg
- 2 tablespoons basil, chopped

Directions:

1. In a bowl, mix the flour, salt, Parmesan, stevia, baking soda, and baking powder and stir.
2. Add the rest of the ingredients gradually and stir the dough well.

3. Transfer it to a lined loaf pan, cook at 350 °F for 1 hour, cool down, slice, and serve.

Nutrition:

- Calories: 231
- Fat: 7 g
- Fiber: 2 g
- Carbohydrates: 5 g
- Protein: 7 g

Beed Bread

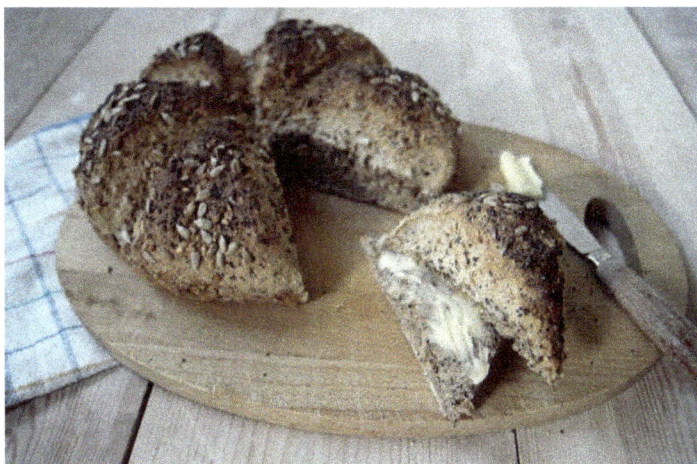

Preparation Time: 1 hour and 10 minutes

Cooking time: 35 minutes

Servings: 6

Ingredients:

- 1 cup warm water
- 3 and ½ cups almond flour
- 1 and ½ cups beet puree
- 2 tablespoons olive oil
- A pinch of salt
- 1 teaspoon stevia
- 1 teaspoon baking powder
- 1 teaspoon baking soda

Directions:

1. In a bowl, mix the flour with the water and beet puree and stir well.
2. Add the rest of the ingredients, stir the dough well and pour it into a lined loaf pan.
3. Leave the mix to rise in a warm place for 1 hour, and then bake the bread at 375 °F for 35 minutes.
4. Cool the bread down, slice, and serve.

Nutrition:

- Calories: 200
- Fat: 8 g
- Fiber: 3 g
- Carbohydrates: 5 g
- Protein: 6 g

Ketogenic Celery Bread

Preparation Time: 2 hours and 10 minutes

Cooking time: 35 minutes

Servings: 6

Ingredients:

- ½ cup celery, chopped
- 3 cups almond flour
- 1 teaspoon baking powder
- 1 teaspoon baking soda
- A pinch of salt
- 2 tablespoons coconut oil, melted
- ½ cup celery puree

Directions:

1. In a bowl, mix the flour with salt, baking powder, and baking soda and stir.
2. Add the rest of the ingredients, stir the dough well, cover the bowl and keep in a warm place for 2 hours.
3. Transfer the dough to a lined loaf pan and cook at 400 °F for 35 minutes.
4. Cool the bread down, slice, and serve.

Nutrition:

- Calories: 162
- Fat: 6 g
- Fiber: 2 g
- Carbohydrates: 6 g
- Protein: 4 g

Easy Cucumber Bread

Preparation Time: 10 minutes
Cooking time: 50 minutes
Servings: 6

Ingredients:

- 1 cup erythritol
- 1 cup coconut oil, melted
- 1 cup almonds, chopped
- 1 teaspoon vanilla extract
- A pinch of salt
- A pinch of nutmeg, ground
- ½ teaspoon baking powder
- A pinch of cloves
- 3 eggs
- 1 teaspoon baking soda
- 1 tablespoon cinnamon powder
- 2 cups cucumber, peeled, deseeded, and shredded
- 3 cups coconut flour
- Cooking spray

Directions:

1. In a bowl, mix the flour with cucumber, cinnamon, baking soda, cloves, baking powder, nutmeg, salt, vanilla extract, and the almonds and stir well.
2. Add the rest of the ingredients except the coconut flour, stir well and transfer the dough to a loaf pan greased with cooking spray.
3. Bake at 325 °F for 50 minutes, cool the bread down, slice, and serve.

Nutrition:

- Calories: 243
- Fat: 12 g
- Fiber: 3 g
- Carbohydrates: 6 g
- Protein: 7 g

Red Bell Pepper Bread

Preparation Time: 10 minutes
Cooking time: 30 minutes
Servings: 12

Ingredients:

- 1 and ½ cups red bell peppers, chopped
- 1 teaspoon baking powder
- 1 teaspoon baking soda
- 2 tablespoons warm water
- 1 and ¼ cups Parmesan, grated
- A pinch of salt
- 4 cups almond flour
- 2 tablespoons ghee, melted
- 1/3 cup almond milk
- 1 egg

Directions:

1. In a bowl, mix the flour with salt, Parmesan, baking powder, baking soda, and bell peppers and stir well.
2. Add the rest of the ingredients and stir the bread batter well.

3. Transfer it to a lined loaf pan and bake at 350 °F for 30 minutes.

4. Cool the bread down, slice, and serve.

Nutrition:

- Calories: 100
- Fat: 5 g
- Fiber: 1 g
- Carbohydrates: 4 g
- Protein: 4 g

Tomato Bread

Preparation Time: 1 hour and 10 minutes

Cooking time: 35 minutes

Servings: 12

Ingredients:

- 6 cups almond flour
- ½ teaspoon basil, dried
- ¼ teaspoon rosemary, dried
- 1 teaspoon oregano, dried
- ½ teaspoon garlic powder
- 2 tablespoons olive oil
- 2 cups tomato juice
- ½ cup tomato sauce
- 1 teaspoon baking powder
- 1 teaspoon baking soda
- 3 tablespoons swerve

Directions:

1. In a bowl, mix the flour with basil, rosemary, oregano, and garlic and stir.
2. Add the rest of the ingredients and stir the batter well.

3. Pour into a lined loaf pan, cover, and keep in a warm place for 1 hour.
4. Bake the bread at 375 °F for 35 minutes, cool down, slice, and serve.

Nutrition:
- Calories: 102
- Fat: 5 g
- Fiber: 3 g
- Carbohydrates: 7 g
- Protein: 4 g

Herbed Ketogenic Bread

Preparation Time: 1 hour and 30 minutes

Cooking time: 40 minutes

Servings: 8

Ingredients:

- 3 cups coconut flour
- 1 teaspoon baking powder
- 1 teaspoon baking soda
- 2 teaspoons stevia
- 1 ½ cups warm water
- ½ teaspoon basil, dried
- 1 teaspoon oregano, dried
- ½ teaspoon thyme, dried
- ½ teaspoon marjoram, dried
- 2 tablespoons olive oil

Directions:

1. In a bowl, mix the flour with baking powder, baking soda, stevia, basil, oregano, thyme, and marjoram and stir.
2. Add the remaining ingredients, mix the dough, cover and keep in a warm place for 1 hour and 30 minutes.

3. Transfer the dough to a floured working surface and knead it again for 2-3 minutes.
4. Transfer to a lined loaf pan and bake at 400 °F for 40 minutes.
5. Cool the bread down before serving.

Nutrition:

- Calories: 200
- Fat: 7 g
- Fiber: 3 g
- Carbohydrates: 5 g
- Protein: 6 g

Green Olive Bread

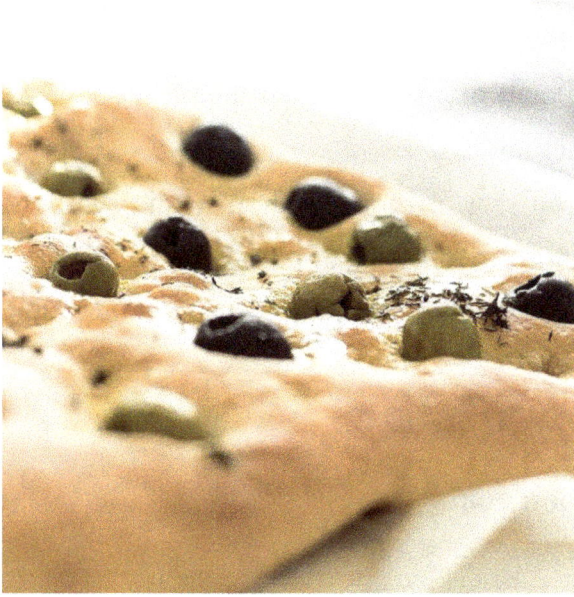

Preparation Time: 10 minutes

Cooking time: 45 minutes

Servings: 10

Ingredients:

- 3 cups almond flour
- A pinch of salt
- ½ teaspoon baking powder
- 1 ½ cups warm water
- 3 tablespoons rosemary, chopped
- ½ cup green olives, pitted and chopped

- A pinch of salt and black pepper

Directions:

1. In a bowl, mix the flour with salt, rosemary, and baking powder and stir.
2. Add the rest of the ingredients, mix the dough well and transfer it to a lined loaf pan.
3. Bake at 400 °F for 45 minutes, cool down, slice, and serve.

Nutrition:

- Calories: 204
- Fat: 12 g
- Fiber: 4 g
- Carbohydrates: 5 g
- Protein: 7 g

Delicious Eggplant Bread

Preparation Time: 10 minutes

Cooking time: 1 hour

Servings: 12

Ingredients:

- 4 eggs, whisked
- 1 cup erythritol
- ½ cup ghee, melted
- ½ cup coconut oil, melted
- 2 cups eggplant, peeled and grated
- 1 tablespoon vanilla extract
- 2 cups almond flour
- 1 ½ teaspoon cinnamon powder
- ¼ teaspoon nutmeg, ground
- ½ teaspoon baking powder
- 1 teaspoon baking soda
- A pinch of salt
- ½ cup pine nuts
- Cooking spray

Directions:

1. In a bowl, mix the flour with cinnamon, nutmeg, baking powder, baking soda, salt, pine nuts, and vanilla and stir.
2. Add the rest of the ingredients except the cooking spray, mix the batter well and pour into a loaf pan greased with the cooking spray.
3. Cook at 350 °F for 1 hour, cool down, slice, and serve.

Nutrition:

- Calories: 200
- Fat: 7 g
- Fiber: 3 g
- Carbohydrates: 5 g
- Protein: 6 g

Great Blackberries Bread

Preparation Time: 10 minutes
Cooking time: 1 hour
Servings: 10

Ingredients:

- 2 cups almond flour
- ½ cup stevia
- 1 ½ teaspoons baking powder
- 1 teaspoon baking soda
- 2 eggs, whisked
- 1 ½ cups almond flour
- ¼ cup ghee, melted
- 1 tablespoon vanilla extract
- 1 cup blackberries, mashed
- Cooking spray

Directions:

1. In a bowl, mix the flour with the baking powder, baking soda, stevia, vanilla, and blackberries and stir well.
2. Add the rest of the ingredients, stir the batter and pour it into a loaf pan greased with cooking spray.
3. Bake at 400 °F for 1 hour, cool down, slice, and serve.

Nutrition:

- Calories: 200
- Fat: 7 g
- Fiber: 3 g
- Carbohydrates: 5 g
- Protein: 7 g

Ketogenic Raspberries Bread

Preparation Time: 10 minutes

Cooking time: 50 minutes

Servings: 6

Ingredients:

- 2 cups almond flour
- 1 teaspoon baking soda
- ¾ cup erythritol
- A pinch of salt
- 1 egg
- ¾ cup coconut milk
- ¼ cup ghee, melted
- 2 cups raspberries
- 2 teaspoons vanilla extract
- ¼ cup coconut oil, melted

Directions:

1. In a bowl, mix the flour with the baking soda, erythritol, salt, vanilla, and raspberries and stir.
2. Add the rest of the ingredients gradually and mix the batter well.

3. Pour this into a lined loaf pan and bake at 350 °F for 50 minutes.
4. Cool the bread down, slice, and serve.

Nutrition:

- Calories: 200
- Fat: 7 g
- Fiber: 3 g
- Carbohidrates: 5 g
- Protein: 7 g

Simple Strawberry Bread

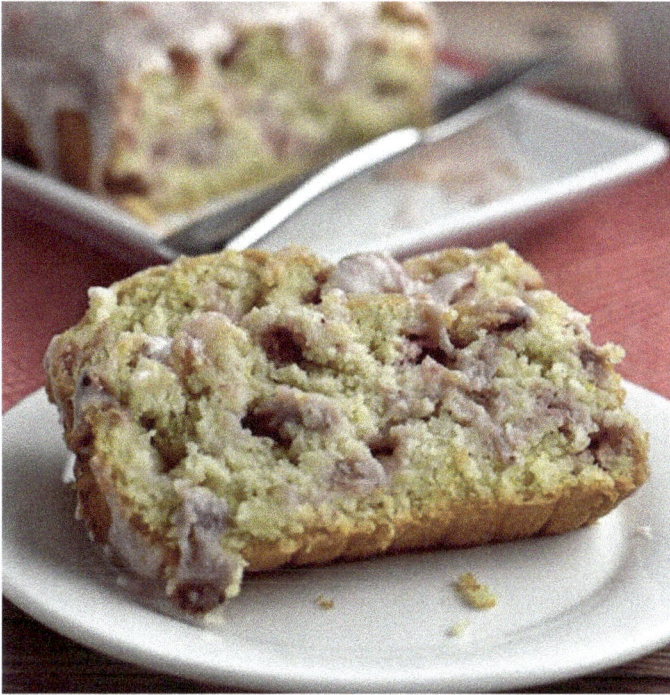

Preparation Time: 10 minutes

Cooking time: 50 minutes

Servings: 8

Ingredients:

- 3 and ½ cups almond flour
- 2 cups strawberries, chopped
- 1 teaspoon baking soda
- 2 cups swerve

- 1 tablespoon cinnamon powder
- 4 eggs, whisked
- 1 ¼ cups coconut oil, melted
- Cooking spray

Directions:

1. In a bowl, mix the flour with baking soda, swerve, strawberries, and cinnamon, and stir.
2. Add the remaining ingredients, stir the batter and pour this into 2 loaf pans greased with cooking spray.
3. Bake at 350 °F for 50 minutes, cool the bread down, slice, and serve.

Nutrition:

- Calories: 221
- Fat: 7 g
- Fiber: 4 g
- Carbohydrates: 5 g
- Protein: 3 g

Great Plum Bread

Preparation Time: 10 minutes

Cooking time: 50 minutes

Servings: 8

Ingredients:

- 1 cup plums, pitted and chopped
- 1½ cups coconut flour
- ¼ teaspoon baking soda
- ½ cup ghee, melted
- A pinch of salt
- 1¼ cups swerve
- ½ teaspoon vanilla extract
- 1/3 cup coconut cream
- 2 eggs, whisked

Directions:

1. In a bowl, mix the flour with baking soda, salt, swerve, and vanilla and stir.
2. In a separate bowl, mix the plums with the remaining ingredients and stir.
3. Combine the 2 mixtures and stir the batter well.

4. Pour into 2 lined loaf pans and bake at 350 °F for 50 minutes.
5. Cool the bread down, slice, and serve them.

Nutrition:
- Calories: 199
- Fat: 8 g
- Fiber: 3 g
- Carbphidrates: 6 g
- Protein: 4 g

Herb Bread

Preparation Time: 1 hour 20 minutes

Cooking Time: 50 minutes (20+30 minutes)

Servings: 1 loaf

Ingredients:

- 3/4 to 7/8 cup milk
- 1 tablespoon sugar
- 1 teaspoon salt
- 1 tablespoon butter or margarine
- 1/3 cup chopped onion
- 2 cups bread flour
- 1/2 teaspoon dried dill
- 1/2 teaspoon dried basil
- 1/2 teaspoon dried rosemary
- 1 ½ teaspoon active dry yeast

Directions:

1. Place all the Ingredients in the bread pan. Select medium crus then the rapid bake cycle. Press starts.

2. After 5-10 minutes, observe the dough as it kneads, if you hear straining sounds in your machine or if the dough appears stiff and dry, add 1 tablespoon Liquid at a time

until the dough becomes smooth, pliable, soft, and slightly tacky to the touch.

3. Remove the bread from the pan after baking. Place on rack and allow to cool for 1 hour before slicing.

Nutrition:

- Calories: 165
- Fat: 5 g
- Carbohydrates: 13 g
- Protein: 2 g

Rosemary Bread

Preparation Time: 2 hours 10 minutes

Cooking Time: 50 minutes

Servings: 1 loaf

Ingredients:

- ¾ cup + 1 tablespoon water at 80 degrees F
- 1 2/3 tablespoons melted butter, cooled
- 1 ½ easpoons sugar
- 1 teaspoon salt
- 1 tablespoon fresh rosemary, chopped
- 2 cups white bread flour
- 1⅓ teaspoons instant yeast

Directions:

1. Add all of the ingredients to your bread machine, carefully following the instructions of the manufacturer.
2. Set the program of your bread machine to Basic/White Bread and set crust type to Medium.
3. Press START.
4. Wait until the cycle completes.
5. Once the loaf is ready, take the bucket out and let the loaf cool for 5 minutes.

6. Gently shake the bucket to remove the loaf.

7. Transfer to a cooling rack, slice, and serve.

Nutrition:

- Calories: 152
- Fat: 3 g
- Carbohydrates: 25 g
- Protein: 4 g
- Fiber: 1 g

Original Italian Herb Bread

Preparation Time: 2 hours 40 minutes

Cooking Time: 50 minutes

Servings: 2 loaves

Ingredients:

- 1 cup water at 80 degrees F
- ½ cup olive brine
- 1½ tablespoons butter
- 1 tablespoons sugar
- 1 teaspoons salt
- 5⅓ cups flour
- 1 teaspoons bread machine yeast
- 20 olives, black/green
- 1½ teaspoons Italian herbs

Directions:

1. Cut olives into slices.
2. Add all of the ingredients to your bread machine (except olives), carefully following the instructions of the manufacturer.
3. Set the program of your bread machine to French bread and set crust type to Medium.

4. Press START.
5. Once the maker beeps, add olives.
6. Wait until the cycle completes.
7. Once the loaf is ready, take the bucket out and let the loaf cool for 5 minutes.
8. Gently shake the bucket to remove the loaf.
9. Transfer to a cooling rack, slice, and serve.

Nutrition:

- Calories: 286
- Fat: 7 g
- Carbohydrates: 61 g
- Protein: 10 g
- Fiber: 1 g

Lovely Aromatic Lavender Bread

Preparation Time: 2 hours 10 minutes

Cooking Time: 50 minutes

Servings: 1 loaf

Ingredients:

- ¾ cup milk at 80 degrees F
- 1 tablespoon melted butter, cooled
- 1 tablespoon sugar
- ¾ teaspoon salt
- 1 teaspoon fresh lavender flower, chopped
- ¼ teaspoon lemon zest
- ¼ teaspoon fresh thyme, chopped
- 1 cups white bread flour
- ¾ teaspoon instant yeast

Directions:

1. Add all of the ingredients to your bread machine
2. Set the program of your bread machine to Basic/White Bread and set crust type to Medium.
3. Press START.
4. Wait until the cycle completes.

5. Once the loaf is ready, take the bucket out and let the loaf cool for 5 minutes.
6. Gently shake the bucket to remove the loaf.
7. Transfer to a cooling rack, slice, and serve.

Nutrition:

- Calories: 144
- Fat: 2 g
- Carbohydrates: 27 g
- Protein: 4 g
- Fiber: 1 g

Oregano Mozza-Cheese Bread

Preparation Time: 2 hours 50 minutes

Cooking Time: 50 minutes

Servings: 2 loaves

Ingredients:

- 1 cup (milk + egg) mixture
- ½ cup mozzarella cheese
- 2¼ cups flour
- ¾ cup whole grain flour
- 1 tablespoon sugar
- 1 teaspoon salt
- 1 teaspoon oregano
- 1½ teaspoons dry yeast

Directions:

1. Add all of the ingredients to your bread machine
2. Set the program of your bread machine to Basic/White Bread and set crust type to Dark.
3. Press START.
4. Wait until the cycle completes.
5. Once the loaf is ready, take the bucket out and let the loaf cool for 5 minutes.

6. Gently shake the bucket to remove the loaf.

7. Transfer to a cooling rack, slice, and serve.

Nutrition:

- Calories: 209
- Fat: 2.1 g
- Carbohydrates: 40 g
- Protein: 7.7 g
- Fiber: 1 g

Cumin Bread

Preparation Time: 3 hours 30 minutes
Cooking Time: 15 minutes
Servings: 8

Ingredients:

- 1 1/3 cups bread machine flour, sifted
- 1½ teaspoons kosher salt
- 1½ tablespoon sugar
- 1 tablespoon bread machine yeast
- 1¾ cups lukewarm water
- 1 tablespoon black cumin
- 1 tablespoon sunflower oil

Directions:

1. Place all the dry and liquid ingredients in the pan and follow the instructions for your bread machine.
2. Set the baking program to BASIC and the crust type to MEDIUM.
3. If the dough is too dense or too wet, adjust the amount of flour and liquid in the recipe.

4. When the program has ended, take the pan out of the bread machine and let it cool for 5 minutes.
5. Shake the loaf out of the pan. If necessary, use a spatula.
6. Wrap the bread with a kitchen towel and set it aside for an hour. Otherwise, you can cool it on a wire rack.

Nutrition:

- Calories: 368
- Total Carbohydrate: 63 g
- Cholesterol: 0 mg
- Total Fat: 6.5 g
- Protein: 9.5 g
- Sodium: 444 mg
- Sugar: 2.5 g

Saffron Tomato Bread

Preparation Time: 3 hours 30 minutes
Cooking Time: 15 minutes
Servings: 10

Ingredients:

- 1 teaspoon bread machine yeast
- 2½ cups wheat bread machine flour
- 1 tablespoon panifarin
- 1½ teaspoons kosher salt
- 1½ tablespoons white sugar
- 1 tablespoon extra-virgin olive oil
- 1 tablespoon tomatoes, dried and chopped
- 1 tablespoon tomato paste
- ½ cup firm cheese (cubes)
- ½ cup feta cheese
- 1 pinch saffron
- 1½ cups serum

Directions:

1. Five minutes before cooking, pour in dried tomatoes and 1 tablespoon of olive oil. Add the tomato paste and mix.

2. Place all the dry and liquid ingredients, except additives, in the pan and follow the instructions for your bread machine.

3. Pay particular attention to measuring the ingredients. Use a measuring cup, measuring spoon, and kitchen scales to do so.

4. Set the baking program to BASIC and the crust type to MEDIUM.

5. Add the additives after the beep or place them in the dispenser of the bread machine.

6. Shake the loaf out of the pan. If necessary, use a spatula.

7. Wrap the bread with a kitchen towel and set it aside for an hour. Otherwise, you can cool it on a wire rack.

Nutrition:

- Calories: 260
- Total Carbohydrates: 33 g
- Cholesterol: 20 g
- Total Fat: 9.2g
- Protein: 8.9 g
- Sodium: 611 mg
- Sugar: 5.2 g

Cracked Black Pepper Bread

Preparation Time: 3 hours 30 minutes
Cooking Time: 15 minutes
Servings: 8

Ingredients:

- ¾ cup water, at 80°F to 90°F
- 1 tablespoon melted butter, cooled
- 1 tablespoon sugar
- ¾ teaspoon salt
- 1 tablespoon skim milk powder
- 1 tablespoon minced chives
- ½ teaspoon garlic powder
- ½ teaspoon cracked black pepper
- 2 cups white bread flour
- ¾ teaspoon bread machine or instant yeast

Directions:

1. Place the ingredients in your bread machine as recommended by the manufacturer.
2. Program the machine for Basic/White bread, select light or medium crust, and press Start.

3. When the loaf is done, remove the bucket from the machine.

4. Let the loaf cool for 5 minutes.

5. Gently shake the bucket to remove the loaf, and turn it out onto a rack to cool.

Nutrition:

- Calories: 141

- Total Carbohydrates: 27 g

- Total Fat: 2g

- Protein: 4 g

- Sodium: 215 mg

- Fiber: 1 g

Spicy Cajun Bread

Preparation Time: 2 hours

Cooking Time: 15 minutes

Servings: 8

Ingredients:

- ¾ cup water, at 80°F to 90°F
- 1 tablespoon melted butter, cooled
- 1 teaspoon tomato paste
- 1 tablespoon sugar
- 1 teaspoon salt
- 2 tablespoons skim milk powder
- ½ tablespoon Cajun seasoning
- 1/8 teaspoon onion powder
- 2 cups white bread flour
- 1 teaspoon bread machine or instant yeast

Directions:

1. Place the ingredients in your bread machine as recommended by the manufacturer.
2. Program the machine for Basic/White bread, select light or medium crust, and press Start.
3. When the loaf is done, remove the bucket from the machine.

4. Let the loaf cool for 5 minutes.
5. Gently shake the bucket to remove the loaf, and turn it out onto a rack to cool.

Nutrition:

- Calories: 141
- Total Carbohydrate: 27 g
- Total Fat: 2g
- Protein: 4 g
- Sodium: 215 mg
- Fiber: 1 g

Anise Lemon Bread

Preparation Time: 2 hours

Cooking Time: 15 minutes

Servings: 8

Ingredients:

- 2/3 cup water, at 80°F to 90°F
- 1 egg, at room temperature
- 2 2/3 tablespoons butter, melted and cooled
- 2 2/3 tablespoons honey
- ⅓ teaspoon salt
- 2/3 teaspoon anise seed
- 2/3 teaspoon lemon zest
- 2 cups white bread flour
- 1⅓ teaspoons bread machine or instant yeast

Directions:

1. Place the ingredients in your bread machine as recommended by the manufacturer.
2. Program the machine for Basic/White bread, select light or medium crust, and press Start.
3. When the loaf is done, remove the bucket from the machine.

4. Let the loaf cool for 5 minutes.

5. Gently shake the bucket to remove the loaf, and turn it out onto a rack to cool.

Nutrition:

- Calories: 158

- Total Carbohydrates: 27 g

- Total Fat: 5g

- Protein: 4 g

- Sodium: 131 mg

- Fiber: 1 g

Cardamon Bread

Preparation Time: 2 hours

Cooking Time: 15 minutes

Servings: 8

- **Ingredients:**
- ½ cup milk, at 80°F to 90°F
- 1 egg, at room temperature
- 1 teaspoon melted butter, cooled
- 1 teaspoon honey
- 2/3 teaspoon salt
- 2/3 teaspoon ground cardamom
- 2 cups white bread flour
- ¾ teaspoon bread machine or instant yeast

Directions:

1. Place the ingredients in your bread machine as recommended by the manufacturer.
2. Program the machine for Basic/White bread, select light or medium crust, and press Start.
3. When the loaf is done, remove the bucket from the machine.
4. Let the loaf cool for 5 minutes.

5. Gently shake the bucket to remove the loaf, and turn it out onto a rack to cool.

Nutrition:

- Calories: 149

- Total Carbohydrates: 29 g

- Total Fat: 2g

- Protein: 5 g

- Sodium: 211 mg

- Fiber: 1 g

Breakfast Bread

Preparation Time: 15 minutes

Cooking Time: 40 minutes

Servings: 16 slices

Ingredients:

- ½ teaspoon. Xanthan gum
- ½ teaspoon. salt
- 2 tablespoons coconut oil
- ½ cup butter, melted
- 1 teaspoon baking powder
- 2 cups of almond flour
- Seven eggs

Directions:

1. Preheat the oven to 355F.
2. Beat eggs in a bowl on high for 2 minutes.
3. Add coconut oil and butter to the eggs and continue to beat.
4. Line a pan with baking paper and then pour the beaten eggs.
5. Pour in the rest of the ingredients and mix until it becomes thick.

6. Bake until a toothpick comes out dry. It takes 40 to 45 minutes.

Nutrition:
- Calories: 234
- Fat: 23 g
- Carbohydrates: 1 g
- Protein: 7 g

Peanut Butter and Jelly Bread

Preparation Time: 2 hours

Cooking Time: 1 hour and 10 minutes

Servings: 1 loaf

Ingredients:

- 1 ½ tablespoons vegetable oil
- 1 cup of water
- ½ cup blackberry jelly
- ½ cup peanut butter
- 1 teaspoon salt
- 1 tablespoon white sugar
- 2 cups of bread flour
- 1 cup whole-wheat flour
- 1 ½ teaspoons active dry yeast

Directions:

1. Put everything in your bread machine pan.
2. Select the basic setting.
3. Press the start button. Take out the pan
4. when done and set it aside for 10 minutes.

Nutrition:

- Calories: 153
- Carbohydrates: 20 g
- Fat: 9 g
- Cholesterol: 0 mg
- Protein: 4 g
- Fiber: 2 g
- Sugar: 11 g
- Sodium: 244 mg
- Potassium: 120 mg

Butter Bread Rolls

Preparation Time: 50 minutes

Cooking Time: 45 minutes

Servings: 24 rolls

Ingredients:

- 1 cup warm milk
- 1/2 cup butter or 1/2 cup margarine, softened
- 1/4 cup sugar
- 2 eggs
- 1 ½ teaspoons salt
- 4 cups bread flour
- 2 ¼ teaspoons active dry yeast

Directions:

1. In the bread machine pan, put all ingredients in the order suggested by the manufacturer.

2. Select dough setting.

3. When the cycle is completed, turn the dough onto a lightly floured surface.

4. Divide dough into 24 portions.

5. Shape dough into balls.

6. Place in a greased 13 inch by a 9-inch baking pan.

7. Cover and let rise in a warm place for 30-45 minutes.

8. Bake at 350 degrees for 13-16 minutes or until golden brown.

Nutrition:

- Carbohydrates: 38 g
- Fat: 2 g
- Protein: 4 g
- Calories: 180

Buttermilk Honey Bread

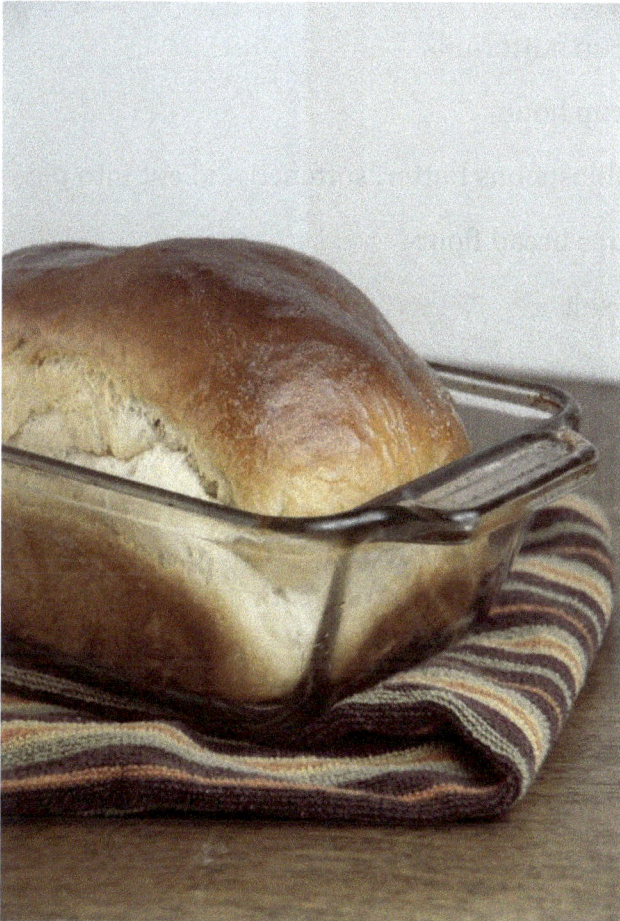

Preparation Time: 5 minutes

Cooking Time: 3 hours 45 minutes

Servings: 14

Ingredients:

- ½ cup water
- ¾ cup buttermilk
- ¼ cup honey
- 3 tablespoons butter, softened and cut into pieces
- 3 cups bread flour
- 1½ salt
- 2¼ teaspoons yeast (or 1 package)

Directions:

1. Add each ingredient to the bread machine in the order and at the temperature recommended by your bread machine man

2. ufacturer. Close the lid, select the basic bread, medium crust setting on your bread machine, and press start. When the bread machine has finished baking, remove the bread and put it on a cooling rack.

Nutrition:

- Carbohydrates: 19 g
- Fat: 1 g
- Protein: 2 g
- Calories: 142

Cranberry Orange Breakfast Bread

Preparation Time: 5 minutes

Cooking Time: 3 hours 10 minutes

Servings: 14

Ingredients:

- 1 1/8 cups orange juice
- 2 tablespoons vegetable oil
- 2 tablespoons honey
- 3 cups bread flour
- 1 tablespoon dry milk powder
- ½ teaspoon ground cinnamon
- ½ teaspoon ground allspice
- 1 teaspoon salt
- 1 (.25 ounce) package active dry yeast
- 1 tablespoon grated orange zest
- 1 cup sweetened dried cranberries
- 1/3 cup chopped walnuts

Directions:

1. Add each ingredient to the bread machine in the order and at the temperature recommended by your bread machine manufacturer.

2. Close the lid, select the basic bread, low crust setting on your bread machine, and press start.

3. Add the cranberries and chopped walnuts 5 to 10 minutes before the last kneading cycle ends.

4. When the bread machine has finished baking, remove the bread and put it on a cooling rack.

Nutrition:

- Carbohydrates: 29 g
- Fat: 2 g
- Protein: 9 g
- Calories: 156

www.ingramcontent.com/pod-product-compliance
Lightning Source LLC
Chambersburg PA
CBHW050747030426
42336CB00012B/1697